IDEA WAYS TO ENLARGE YOUR PENIS 100% ORGANICALLY.

Discovering the natural ways to penis enlargement.

By

Dr DOUGLAS JASON

TABLE OF CONTENTS

ABOUT THE AUTHOR

INTRODUCTION.

TABLE OF CONTENTS

ABOUT THE AUTHOR

Dr DOUGLAS JASON is a certified dietician who has a strong passion for wellness and a big eagerness to help people all over the world. He uses healthy food, herbs, sauce and other useful tools to help mankind realized it's overall goal of optimum health.

Introduction:

For many individuals across the globe, the size of the penis has been a source of intrigue and worry. Although there are several techniques and items on the market that promise to expand the penis, there is rising enthusiasm for discovering organic, natural, and secure solutions to accomplish this objective. This thorough manual will look at 10 distinct theories and techniques that could help expand the penis naturally, without the use of artificial substances or intrusive surgeries. We will go into each strategy in depth, including explanations, examples, and insights on their effectiveness and safety. These approaches range from lifestyle modifications to workouts, herbal cures, and more.

CHAPTER 1

Healthy Lifestyle Options.

Sexual health is only one aspect of total well-being that may be greatly influenced by a healthy lifestyle. The emphasis of this chapter will be on how adopting a healthy lifestyle might perhaps aid in penis growth attempts. We will go through the significance of eating a balanced diet, getting regular exercise, controlling stress, getting enough sleep, abstaining from smoking and binge drinking alcohol, and drinking enough water. There will be examples of various meals, workouts, and relaxation methods

that might promote penile health
and perhaps help with enlargement.

CHAPTER 2

Exercises for the penis.

Pelvic floor exercises, often known as kegel exercises, are a variety of exercises that concentrate on the muscles around and around the penis. This chapter explains how these workouts might strengthen muscles, boost blood flow, and perhaps result in a gradual increase in size. We will go through the proper way to conduct kegel exercises, provide instances of many kegel variants, and go over the advantages and disadvantages of including them in a regular regimen.

CHAPTER 3

herbal remedies.

Traditional medicine has long employed herbal medicines to treat a range of ailments, including sexual wellness. This chapter will examine many herbs, including tribulus terrestris, ginseng, and ginkgo biloba, which are thought to have potential penis enlarging qualities. We will discuss the use of these herbs, their possible advantages, and any known hazards or safety measures related to their usage. We'll talk about a few herbal pills, drinks, and topical remedies that might promote penile growth.

CHAPTER 4

Manual stretching techniques.

The penile tissue may be stretched manually by gently pushing or stroking it with the hands. This chapter will discuss several manual stretching methods, including jelqing and stretching exercises, and how they may help enlarge the penis. We'll go through how to do it step-by-step, what to watch out for, and any possible advantages of adding manual stretching exercises to a penile growth regimen. There will be demonstrations of appropriate approaches and variants.

CHAPTER 5

Devices Using Vacuum.

Penis pumps, which mechanically produce a vacuum around the penis to suck blood into the erectile chambers and maybe encourage greater growth, are sometimes referred to as vacuum devices. This chapter will cover the operation of vacuum devices, as well as any possible advantages and use dangers. We'll talk about various vacuum gadgets, such as manual and electric pumps, and provide examples of how to use them properly and avoid dangerous situations.

Chapter 6:

Body Fat Reduction and Weight Loss.

The penis may look smaller than it is due to excess body fat, especially in the pubic region. In the context of penis enlargement, this chapter will emphasize the possible advantages of weight loss and body fat reduction. We will talk about how adopting a healthy lifestyle that includes exercise and weight loss may enhance penis size. Examples of effective activities, food adjustments, and weight loss and body fat reduction techniques will be given.

Chapter 7

Discusses psychological factors and mindfulness.

Sexual health and the sense of penis size may be impacted by psychological variables such as stress, anxiety, and body image problems.
By enhancing general sexual health and self-confidence, mindfulness techniques and psychological issues may help with penile growth. To promote the aims of penis expansion, we will provide examples of mindfulness practices, stress-reduction methods, and ways to create a good body image.

CHAPTER 8

Adequate Sleep and Hormonal Balance.

Hormonal balance and general health are both greatly influenced by sleep. The relationship between sufficient sleep and hormonal balance in penile expansion will be discussed in this chapter. We will talk about how penis size and sexual health may be impacted by hormonal abnormalities, such as low testosterone levels. We'll also stress how crucial it is to obtain enough good sleep to maintain hormonal harmony and possible penile development. Examples of lifestyle

modifications, sleep hygiene
techniques, and hormonal support
techniques will be given.

CHAPTER 9

Massage and Circulation.

Techniques for massaging the body might perhaps help with penile expansion by increasing blood flow and encouraging the formation of healthy tissue. The many massage treatments covered in this chapter, including lymphatic massage, penile enlargement massage, and others, may assist to improve blood flow to the penis and maybe encourage size improvements. We will outline the specific procedures, safety warnings, and possible advantages of including massage in a penile growth regimen. There will be

examples of appropriate massage
methods and variations.

CHAPTER 10

Patience and Consistency.

Any attempt to grow the penis requires patience and persistence. This chapter will stress the need of having a realistic outlook and stay committed to the tactics you have selected throughout time. We'll talk about how penis expansion is a progressive process that calls for commitment, tolerance, and perseverance. Along the way, we'll provide advice on how to monitor our progress, establish reasonable goals, and maintain our motivation. We'll provide you with some real-life success tales and testimonies from people who, with persistence and patience, grew their penis naturally.

CONCLUSION

The idea of naturally and organically enlarging the penis has attracted a lot of interest. A healthcare expert should always be consulted before making any modifications, even though there are many ideas and approaches accessible. In this comprehensive guide, we've covered ten concepts, including healthy lifestyle choices, penis exercises, herbal remedies, manual stretching techniques, vacuum devices, weight loss and body fat reduction, mindfulness, and psychological factors, sufficient sleep and hormonal balance, massage and circulation, the value of patience and consistency, and weight loss and body fat reduction. Each strategy offers possible advantages, dangers, and safety measures, and outcomes may change depending on the person. It's critical to keep in mind that communication with partners and confidence are crucial components of a successful sexual relationship and that penis size is not the only indicator of sexual health or masculinity. It could be feasible to accomplish organic penile growth safely and healthily with the appropriate technique, patience, and persistence.